My Tea Taste Much Better

My Tea Taste Much Better

How to generate positive emotional frequencies, Manage Stress, and live a happier, healthier life

R. Jean Johnson, M.Ed.

Beaconwear Books

Library of Congress Control Number:

2024925376

ISBN: 979-8-218-55914-4

Publisher: Beaconwear Books

Email: beaconwearbooks@gmail.com

R. Jean Johnson, M.Ed.

My Tea Taste Much Better

1: Mind and body healing, 2: Self-management,

3: Psychology, 4: Body-sculpting

Dedication

This book is dedicated to people everywhere who are trying to live their best life! To get the most out of this resource, please suspend your tendency to compare, skip over sections, because you think you know. You don't know. This book was written from a totally different perspective, one that you've never encountered before. So, approach this book as you would a class on a subject you may have heard of, but know nothing about; then, you'll realize the full benefit of the experiences, information, and strategies I offer you.

Table of Contents

Preface

The idea to write *My Tea Taste Much Better* was serendipitous. I had been dealing with a couple of persistent life challenges that had become overwhelming; and it became clear something had to give. Either I was going to keep stressing over these issues, or I was going to leave them to the Divine course of the universe to resolve; because my daily anxiety was getting me nowhere. So, I decided to go with the latter: leave the result to a higher power. I stopped stressing; ruminating, scratching my head, and demanding that other people do thus-and-so to rid me of these problems; and 'lo and behold,' something happened that I'd not experienced in decades – Peace! I felt a peace that I had forgotten was even possible. Then, something more wonderful occurred – my daily cup of tea tasted phenomenal! It was as though I was drinking tea for the first time, and never knew how fantastic of an experience it could be. That's when I had an Epiphany: Our senses (taste and so forth) are impacted by our emotions; even our taste buds suffer when we subject ourselves to prolonged stress. Mental health experts like David Arterburn, M.D. of Kaiser Permanente, and Washington Health Research Institute, states, "Mood disorders may lead to weight gain – and vice versa. Some people use eating as a coping mechanism for sadness, because certain foods, like refined sugars, can have an opiate-like effect on the brain." This high is only temporary, however.

Relationships present our most difficult challenges. We were taught, at least in Western Society, to depend on others for our very survival. Add to that, the fact, emotionally, we are rarely, if ever, taught that we are separate entities from all other people, though we must live interdependently, on some levels. Had we been taught about our uniqueness, and how we can use our unique skills to forge a life that is meaningful, if separate from others, I believe, we'd have much less mental disorders, anger and violence in Western Society. Hence, we are psychologically- dependent on others for our well-being to the point of mental and emotional imbalance. We must learn to depend more on ourselves and less on others.

Originality is a highly-sustainable life skill that enables us to detach from others when our needs are no longer being met, or the relationship is too difficult to maintain, without going to extremes, like retaliating against those who we perceived hurt, abandoned, or done us some other injustice. I would encourage you to discover yours.

The reality of life is that no one can be all things to all people; and, we are responsible for facing our fears, (however painful or scary); taking control of our emotions, changing bad habits that can lead to mental illness, and believing we are worth all of our efforts. This sounds overwhelming, I know; and, even impossible for many of us, based on the "Hell!" we have suffered; but like the little train that could, we must move along the tracks of our past trauma, little by little, making progress in small increments, until we realize, "I think I can." Hence, due to all of the above, the book you are reading was born.

My hope and prayer, is that *My Tea Taste Much Better* will reduce the stress and worry that plagues your life, allowing you to experience joy and peace at a higher frequency than ever before and lead you to a life *more* worth living, and a first step towards self-sufficiency.

Introduction

The mind is a storage box of our experiences and impressions. Good experiences leave positive impressions and bad experiences the opposite. What is so profound is that bad impressions can linger, not only in your mind as thoughts, but also in your body as *vibrations*. These vibrations (which vibrate at certain frequencies) can impact your feelings and other senses, as well. This book will delve into how your senses: taste, smell, and the like, are altered by your emotions; and what you can do to enhance those vibrations such that your senses operate at their highest (positive) frequency; thus providing you with the most enjoyable manifestation of each of your senses and improve your overall health. Remember, the key to a journey of a thousand miles is taking the first step.

Our body functions are controlled by a complex system of interactions between various glands, the hormones they produce, and cells. Depending on whether this system is working in harmony (or not) determines if the frequency of the vibrations (in your body tissues and muscles, etc.) produce positive or negative outcomes. It seems simple to think that we can easily control these vibrational effects; if we just discipline our thoughts. Unfortunately, nothing could be further from the truth. The fact is hormones have such a powerful impact on our minds that we must employ a variety of strategies to train (identify and respond to the vibrations we experience) our bodies and minds to practice positive habits; thereby increasing the positive vibrations (or frequencies), so we can counter-act the devastating effects stress can have on our health, life and relationships.

Another way to explain the impact hormones have on your body is to use the term, impulses. When you think about impulses, like the desire to smoke a cigarette, or have a glass of wine; these "cravings," if you will, start with a strong feeling (vibration) within the body; though they feel as though they are being generated by the mind. Now, as the desires get stronger, the vibration(s) also become more intense (vibrate at a lower, but intense frequency), and unless something is done to intercept and moderate these vibrations, you will find yourself smoking cigarettes, or drinking several glasses of wine. When the body is under such extreme stress, normal cravings can become self-destructive habits. As a result of impulses, such as cravings for foods or other substances that are not good for us, in high amounts, stress hormones are released in our brain, flowing to various cells in our bodies, (potentially) wreaking havoc on our senses, depending on our state of mind. This leads to either over (or under) stimulated cells, such as our taste buds; resulting in overeating, drinking, or excess worry. In the case of under stimulation, we may fall into a catatonic-like state, where we under-respond to stimuli, i.e. complete loss of appetite, which can result in dangerous weight loss. These hormone imbalances can rise to dangerous levels. As a result, a state of mental and or physical sickness (imbalance) or disease can ensue. This *out-of-balance* hormonal state must be brought back into balance (recalibrated) in order to regain our health and well-being. Thus, vibrations are those forces within us that are so strong that unless a *force equal or greater than* the vibration, counteracts the intensity of the "impulses," you will be hopelessly at the mercy of these powerful internal mind and body forces. This is the reason many of you find it so hard to break habits that seem to hold you hostage. The goal of *My Tea Taste Much Better* is to provide you with a guide, some insights, and strategies to outsmart (or lessen) those vibrational pulls that keep you going left, when you want (and need) to go right, helping you to achieve greater mental and emotional balance.

To set the stage for our discussion, going forward, about how the body is impacted by powerful hormones, I want to give you context. The main culprit is cortisol. It regulates every other function within the body. So, to just give you a brief summary as you read on, this is what the powerful hormone, cortisol controls, and how it causes our organs, and cells to operate correctly, or not, inside the human body:

More specifically, cortisol affects your body in the following ways:

Regulating your body's stress response:

During times of stress, your body can release cortisol after releasing its "fight or flight" hormones, such as adrenaline, so you continue to stay on high alert. In addition, cortisol triggers the release of glucose (sugar) from your liver for fast energy during times of stress or physical exertion.

Regulating metabolism:

Cortisol helps control how your body uses fats, proteins and carbohydrates for energy.

Suppressing inflammation: Short spurts of cortisol boost your immunity, but if you have consistently high levels of cortisol, it can lead to inflammation and a weakened immune system.

Regulating blood pressure: The exact way in which cortisol regulates blood pressure in humans is unclear. However, elevated levels of cortisol can cause high blood pressure, and lower-than-normal levels of cortisol can cause low blood pressure, both dangerous to your health.

Increasing and regulating blood sugar: Under normal circumstances, cortisol counterbalances the effect of insulin, a hormone your pancreas makes, to regulate your blood sugar. Cortisol raises blood sugar by releasing stored glucose, while insulin lowers blood sugar. Having chronically- high cortisol levels can lead to persistent high blood sugar (hyperglycemia). This can cause Type 2 diabetes. The next function is extremely important.

Helps control your sleep-wake cycle: Under regular

circumstances, you have lower cortisol levels in the evening when you go to sleep and peak levels in the morning right before you wake up. This suggests that cortisol plays a significant role in the initiation of wakefulness and plays a part in your body's circadian rhythm. The above list of cortisol functions comes from the Cleveland Clinic Medical Professional Review, dated 12/10/2021.Thus, the first step in this entire process is being more aware of you. But, that's easier said than done. Thus, self-awareness is the key to learning how you function. This almost seems obvious, but, as I'm sure you will agree, we pay far less attention to what's going on in us than we do to what's going on around us. So, let's start with just paying attention to the most important person in your life – you; because if you're not happy, no one else around you will be. What are you feeling – right now?

AWARENESS

A great sage by the name of Swami Rama stated:

"The purpose and aim of life is to remain in constant awareness of the reality. The whole lamp of life is lighted by that awareness, for it is the source of all knowledge. Awareness is not a thought; it is not an emotion; it is not a desire. But that which inspires thought, the power through which thought functions, the power through which emotions work, the power through

which desires function—that power is called awareness. "

In the Swami's quote, we see that the idea that being in touch with reality is the central requirement to making change. It makes sense; because how can we see the forest, but not the trees? In other words, what we think we see is not always reality. So, the first thing we must do is to see clearly. That's a tall order. People routinely see what they want to see or allow their feelings or desires to dictate their actions, often resulting in disappointment, miscues, and personal loss.

So, how do we start to see what is real? First, ask yourself questions: What am I feeling? Why am I feeling what I'm feeling? Are these feelings rational, or borne out of desire, anger, fear, or loneliness? Hence, identify the truth as it relates to your current situation.

Once you've hashed out the "reality" of what you are feeling, then it will be possible for you to ask yourself the next set of questions: What do I need to do to make this situation I'm dealing with better? Say, you are having sad feelings; and those feelings are causing you to overeat or drink alcohol to excess. You want to be courageous in your acceptance of the reality of your problem(s). This would be a good opportunity to write your feelings down in a journal, and include dates; so you can create sort of a timeline and keep track of your successes in overcoming these issues.

Carl Jung, a great philosopher, said:

"Once you understand your psychological patterns and the negative affect these patterns have on your life, you can now make better life choices. This is a breakthrough!"

To help you figure out where you need to make changes, use some of the following activities whenever you're feeling out-of-sorts, in a rut, afraid, angry, or confused, to develop a more peaceful state of mind.

- **Sleep**: There's a mind-body connection to good overall health. So, let's start at the beginning: You need 7-9 hours (depending on age and sex) per night to function at optimal levels

According to Michael Breus, author of <u>The Sleep Doctor's Diet Plan: Lose</u>

Weight Through Better Sleep, "The consistency of a person's sleep schedule and getting six hours of sleep, or more, a night were two key factors in their ability to lose weight." Thus, restful sleep is critical for a sound mind and body."

Meditation

- Creates calm in your life
- Helps to refocus your thoughts and energies
- Provides a new reason to keep moving forward: i.e. purpose
- Raises self-esteem

- Reminds you that you can start anew even if you're alone for the time being
- Most importantly, it gives you Hope for a better future.

Unclutter your environment

- Sell or donate things you've not used in years
- Garden:

You'll be surprised at how digging your hands into dirt can rejuvenate your spirit. It can be done in or outdoors

Listen to classical music.

- There is ample research that shows listening to classical music calms the mind and improves focus. I use it regularly: While working on projects (school work, to exercise, etc.)

Get creative

Draw, paint, or learn to play an instrument

Travel

- Start local then branch out
- Solo or with others. To help you plan your first trip, order my travel guide, <u>Don't Wait, Celebrate Life! Single</u>

Gals Guide to Traveling Solo, by Rena Johnson, M.Ed.

Meet with a therapist: The **American Psychological Association** is a good resource for references. We all need a little help sometime; so don't feel embarrassed.

Massage Therapy

-Our bodies respond to touch; especially, soft soothing touch. In some cultures, it's offered as part of the mental health practitioner's services to patients

Read

- Mysteries take you out of your life for a moment, and launch you into a world of imagination. This can be very cathartic, as you delve deep into the world of make believe. You may even gain some insight into a new way of thinking that may have a positive impact on your real life.
- Autobiographies: This is one of the best ways to learn how to overcome challenges. Some of our greatest leaders had to face major difficulties to become the person they ultimately became.

Whether you engage in listening to music, take an art or architecture class, learning about how to re-imagine your problems can help you think about your challenges more creatively.

Monitor your thinking

- How do you think, generally? Do you find yourself scrutinizing everything and everybody for the smallest discrepancy? Then, do you judge that decrepancy like it was the plague? If so, this is very, very bad. I know for a fact it is, because this is one of my problems. And, let me tell you, it gets so tiresome. What can we do to stop this negative mental trait?

- Use a word like "Stop!" to say to yourself silently, or out loud, if no ones around, to intercept that thought.
- Read some bible verses on how not to judge and why you shouldn't
- Keep a small notebook with you and every time

you start judging, notate it.

- If you have a trusted confidant, call them and let them know you're at it again. And, invite them to coffee to discuss how this bad habit is ruining your peace of mind. Maybe they'll be smpathetic and provide support.
- Write a "letter to self." State how anxious and fearful, judging others

makes you feel. And, vow
to not judge anyone for
the next hour.

These kinds of simple, but effective actions can began to help loosen the grip that negative mindsets, and the behavior traits that accompany them, have on your thinking, and actions; and how to change them to more positive thoughts and actions.

Eat slowly and monitor when you're satisfied: According to Dr. Karen Grothe, of the Mayo Clinic: We eat without thought, as though it's just another task. It takes 20-30 minutes before our brain is signaled, that we're full.

PERCEPTION

I was sitting on my veranda, recently, just enjoying a cup of tea (ironic huh?), and my mind was just wandering from thought to thought, and sight to sight. Suddenly, my eyes veered downward, for some reason, and there it was. Not three feet from where I sat, was this frog. Now, you might say: What's the big deal? Well, I live in an urban area, and in the nearly twenty years I've lived in this particular area, I'd never seen anything more than a small tadpole, in a stream or creek. To see this palm-sized frog, sitting on my porch, was exciting, and at the same time – curious. Moreover, I wondered how long it'd been sitting there, (waiting for me to notice it–☺); and why I hadn't spotted it sooner? I understand better now.

We see what we focus on, or favor. What? Our perception is based on a bias of our own personal preference. So, just like I saw the morning doves, cardinals, the gold and brown leaves falling off the trees, and cars racing back and forth on my street, I did not choose to see what was right there in front of me. What a revelation! When it's put that way, it can feel a little unsettling, can't it? Clear perception is not only necessary to manage our emotions; it can also be a life-saver. What if that frog had been a poisonous snake? Ergo, developing your ability to perceive – rightly, is a valuable life skill in learning *what is vs personal* biases. How many times have you ignored the obvious, and regretted it? I bet you're thinking – "Wow, if only I'd paid better attention to that last conversation I had with 'so and so,' it would have made all the difference in our relationship. We might even still be friends. I really missed out on a great friendship." Or, your regret could be on another subject all together, but no doubt, you, like all of us, regret what we ignored.

That whole little whimsical story I just shared with you about the frog, was to prepare you for the truth of how the human mind is capable of setting us up for success or failure – depending on how we choose to "perceive" things. If anyone can attest to this fact, it's me. I've allowed my flawed-perception to get me into so many tight places, that if I had a dollar …….; well, you know the rest. But, alas, as the Good Book says: God works in mysterious ways. Hence,

I would have never been able to share these truths with you, if I had not experienced them for myself? So, the universe is working according to plan. So, let's get down to business. Understanding more about how your body (and mind) works is paramount to gaining control over your emotions. The truth is, most of us have damaged emotions, and we have created, in our minds, ways of coping; but these unrealistic coping skills only mask the pain we feel. We must bring the pain of our traumatized emotions to the fore to change how we feel and behave when triggered.

The problem, as stated by Carl Jung, one of the greatest philosophers of the 20th Century:

"Those patterns have kept you stuck from living the life you have imagined. Of course, your experiences and the way you coped with them will never disappear. They are part of your spiritual development. However, the coping mechanisms and false beliefs are no longer dictating who you become, your authentic self, the self that wants purpose and meaning in life." **(*The Collected Works of Carl Jung*, Vol. 11, Para 391)**

I've told you how over or under stimulated cells, can sabotage our senses. This imbalance occurs when our adrenal gland sends out too much cortisol: (increased vibrations at higher frequencies than normal), of a hormone, like Glucocorticoids, into the bloodstream. This over/under stimulation can result in conditions such as depression, insomnia, or anxiety; which can lead to overeating, or other adverse behaviors. In fact, according to Bradley Nelson, DC (doctor of Chiropractic), *"trapped Emotional vibrations*" causes surrounding tissues (cells) to vibrate at the same frequency, known as resonance, (Healthline, September 16, 2021.) Thus, stress can cause our hormones to derail, overwhelm our cells (i.e. taste, brain: amygdala, etc.), and work against our best interests; because they can tell our minds something is true, when it's not: we're hungry, when we're actually scared, tired, or lonely. Our signals get crossed as a result; and, we find ourselves at the mercy of this destructive hormonal-imbalance. The question is: How can we outsmart ourselves? We can't. However, we can play to our strengths: give the enemy (our cravings, anger, or sadness), something similar to what it wants, but not what it wants. For instance, though we can't stop a sweet-binge from coming on, we can give it low-cal hot chocolate, instead of that chocolate cupcake we're pinning for, or a bowl of naturally-sweet pineapple, instead of that bowl of pineapple ice cream. First, we have to train our minds to intercept our out-of-control hormones; by *perceiving* that a craving is coming on; and, at the onset; we can jump into action, using activities and/or strategies to stop them in their tracks! What if we started out each day by perceiving our blessings? Wouldn't this practice set our minds in a positive mode before any hormonal imbalance that might occur during the day has the chance to sabotage our thinking? We can begin to develop a new approach to dealing with our emotional imbalances by recalling those things that we feel good about. Is there anything you're thankful for? Write it down and watch what happens.

(To let you off the hook, sometimes nothing will do, but that scoop of ice cream, or slice of chocolate cake. So, give yourself a break, if you indulge from time to time.) The key is to slowly change how we respond to stressful emotions.)

Gratitude Journal

A gratitude journal can be a fun and creative endeavor, if you just let your imagination flow. For example, pick up an inexpensive notebook from one of those discount stores, along with a few colored pencils, or markers, and maybe a few decorations. Then, let your imagination run wild. Start with a theme: birds, trees, or whatever suits your creative fancy. Next, draw some images representing that theme, cut some from a magazine, or print some from the internet to make your journal uniquely-you. You may also want to carry this theme on to each page in your journal. Once you have your theme in place, take the next steps:

- Each morning, write three things you are grateful for, right now.
- Recite those three things out loud while writing them in your journal
- Throughout the day revisit these items to reinforce these areas of gratitude, especially if something upsetting occurs.

- Use index cards to post what you're grateful for in conspicuous places around your home. If you use erasable ink, you can reuse the cards daily.

This strategy alone can go a long way to combatting the anxiety we all feel. In fact, according to Robert Hudak, MD, in psychiatry, at the University Of Pittsburg Medical Center Western Psychiatric Hospital, "Anxiety disorders are among the most common mental health issues in the United States, with more than 15 percent of adults reporting symptoms of anxiety in

2019." Thus, feeling more gratitude in our daily lives will only lessen our feelings of anxiety, bringing us into a more balanced emotional state. Here are some other ideas to improve your mood and increase gratitude, resulting in more peace and less angst.

Chase the sun

I always feel better when the sun is beaming down on me. Try these ideas for spending more time in the sun. Not only will you get your daily dose of vitamin D, you'll enjoy it!

- Start a daily ritual of getting up at sunrise

- Play music to match that glorious feeling you get when you see that beautiful ball of fire rising "Here comes the sun" comes to mind. You choose your favorite.
- Do ten jumping jacks, or ten minutes on your stationary bike, while watching the sun come up, to get your circulation moving
- Take a sunrise walk. Listening to the sounds of nature is almost meditative; especially when no one else is around to disturb that peace. Soak it all in and begin to heal.

- Buy a pot of sunflowers. So, even when the day is overcast, you'll still have the sun right next to you on your nightstand
- Sit on the porch and watch the sun come up while, what else, having a cup of tea!
- If you have a dog, take it for a sunrise walk. It'll love you for it. If you can, add a slow jog to the mix, you'll both feel better.

There's always something to celebrate. So, pick an occasion and have at it! You'll get just as much out of it as the person for whom you're planning. In the end, less stress, more joy, and a healthier state of mind is the pay off.

Choose satisfying, but nutritional foods, on purpose:

The overwhelming reason why most of us overeat is to get a quick high, especially when we're feeling down. What we don't quite understand is that "high" is generated by another powerful hormone – dopamine. Unfortunately, the foods that give us the greatest charge of dopamine are the ones we like – high caloric, low-nutrition foods. Thus, it is extremely important for us to be "mindful" about not only how we're feeling, and the triggers that accompany those feelings (i.e. sad, mad, frustrated, lonely, etc.), but what foods we can eat, get a feeling of relief, and not do damage to our health. So, foods high in nutrition, that taste good is what we must aim for; so, that when we are triggered by a low-vibrational hormone, i.e. cortisol, in excess, we reach for a treat that will sooth us and maintain our health. Fruit, vegetables, and yogurt are good choices. There are a variety of tasty, yet nutritious foods out there. Do a little research to find the ones best for you.

FORGIVENESS

How do you forgive the unforgivable: people who you should have been able to count on, especially as a child, betrayed you, abandoned you; and on top of all that, they made you feel unworthy? As a result, you trust no one and criticize others just as you were so-badly criticized. This state of mind can lead to a lifetime of trauma, including depression, PTSD, stress and anxiety. The only avenue for healing and freedom is – Forgiveness. This might be forgiving the person(s) whom harmed you, or just forgiving yourself, in the case that the other person(s) is/are no longer around, or refuses to have a conversation about the wrong(s) done to you and that still plague you.

It's a psychological fact that when you feel good about yourself and your life, you are more able to forgive past injustices. Just try it. Do something, healthy and positive, that makes you feel great; and see how much more agreeable you become. Thus, a first step to forgiveness is feeling better about yourself and your life.

To start changing the dynamics of your thinking from resentful to forgiving, try these strategies:

Express your feelings and plan your future

- Self-awareness Journaling
- Be honest with how you "really" feel about those people or circumstances that have traumatized you
- Set goals to put the trauma behind you
  - One year
  - Two year …

By the 3rd year, be ready to release all of the hostility to the wind, and move in a more positive direction

Get creative

- Draw
- Design a mission board
- Write poetry

Start a support group

Sharing a problem is always the best way to move past it; because others who've endured the same struggles may have good ideas on how to overcome the shared problems you face. So, join or start a group.

Reach beyond your immediate environment

Sometimes you have to get *away* to relieve stress; especially if your trauma occurred in the same environment that you currently reside. Nothing gets you out of your head, like a change in scenery.

Travel

- Take a trip to an exotic location
    - Meet new people who may become new friends
- Pretend you're on an adventure
- Treasure hunt

- Sea shell gathering
- Visit historic estates with a mysterious past
- Check out some flea markets

Start a self-help book club

- To keep expenses down, ask members to get books on loan from their local library
- Have a weekly zoom reading
- Charge a small membership fee, so you can have a monthly raffle, giving the book-of-the month as the prize.

ACCEPTANCE

If Forgiveness is hard, Acceptance can be even harder. How can you accept that the time you put into a relationship is gone forever? Or, how can you endure the reality that the trauma that others caused you will prevent you from ever becoming that vision you had of yourself? These truths of life may seem too hard to bear; but bear we must, if we want to move beyond the pain of the past. First, face your pain, with help;

then seek out those authentic parts of yourself and learn to express them.

There certainly will be a cooling-off period, so-to-speak, before we come to the truth of our predicament. It can take years (even decades) to accept, emotionally, what you've long had to grapple with in order to survive. Every day you've had to get up, get dressed, maybe get kids ready for school, and the like, all while bearing a seemingly unbearable pain of loss or betrayal. And, that pain has held you back from the simple joys of life, much less venturing into a new relationship; which at this stage, you've sworn off to ever try again. But, alas, you finally realize that the key to your salvation is to accept life as it is, and move forward with what you have left. That's it! What do you have left? That dream you once had, can you still pursue it, albeit on a different level? What about learning some new skills: a language, art or music? These are all viable options, once you accept that the past is in the past. Remember we can only change the present and potentially the future. So, let's investigate what a "new" you may look like in this new future you're forging.

You've accepted that life rarely goes according to plan; and that you must focus only on that which you can control, not on what is outside the bounds of your control.

The next thing you must do is embrace flexibility in thinking, temper expectations, and execute actions. Nobody's perfect; and trying to be perfect is exhausting and usually leads to extreme frustration. It can even lead to mental illness: depression, neurosis, psychosis, etc. These conditions can be difficult or impossible to overcome. Thus, changing your mindset about perfection, is not only healthy, but can be life-saving! Besides, trying to be perfect is just plain old boring. So, find out who you really are (i.e. what makes you happy and is not self-destructive); and cultivate a life based on your authentic self. Acceptance is simpler than we think if we really look at it in an objective fashion. In fact, you have all the insight and inner tools you need. Just look around you. Everything in life is unique. What this means, is that you aren't made like the next person; duplicating others is futile. So, Carpe diem! Take positive actions borne out of a new sense of positive self-awareness. Don't be afraid to ask for help.

I need to make a comment about anger. It can be a positive force, but history shows it usually results in some kind of violence. But, what if we could reimagine our anger – the power it holds? What if we could take that drive and apply it to something wonderful? For example, restoring some antiques to their original glory. Or, teaching a group of foster kids at the local girls and boys club how to use a computerized drawing application. Who knows, you may discover the next Picasso.

Moving Forward

I remember when people would say to me, “Just move on!” when I’d try to tell them how traumatic my childhood was: how my own mother ruined my emotional health to the point the trauma affected my entire life. So many good things that the universe presented to me were lost due to my inability to navigate the social contract appropriately. Years later, the shear loss and betrayal I endured were so entrenched and intense, they colored every part of my life a dull-gray; and, few, if any, of the people I wanted so desperately to understand me, and feel my pain – could. In fact, they thought I was either nuts, or a cry-baby. That's why their response, "Just move on!" was so debilitating. I felt so alone, most times. When you feel alone, it's hard to move on. It's like a baseball player at bat, but there's no pitcher to pitch the ball to him. How do you proceed? Truth is you can't, until something penetrates that dull-gray layer of pain on your soul, and you realize, as Kenny Loggins so eloquently put it: This is it!

Then, a light comes on. It shines on your *now* – not the past. You come to a hard-stop, telling yourself: I've got to move; where, I don't know, but something has to change, if I'm going to live, at all! So, you pull out your notebook and start figuring out what you have left: talent, interest, desires, skills, hopes, and dreams. You decide on which two or three things, you've listed, are still possible. Then, you make a plan to proceed. It won't be easy, but the key is that you must stop bemoaning your painful past, look to the present, and the possibility of a future that's based on your authentic self. Be patient, too; change takes time. And, when you need to, cry. It's one of the best stress relievers, money can't buy!

Here's the central question, "Who are you now?" Start with what you've been doing over the past 5 years that brings you pleasure. Write down that place you visited or experience you had that made you laugh-out-loud, felt fulfilled; activating old or new dreams of some goal you once vowed to achieve. It may have changed from years ago, but the feeling you get when you remember that thing, is what you want to capture, conceptualize, and devise a plan to bring to life in this "now season" of the *best* of your life. Try things on for size, and then build from there.

Next, figure out if what you want is coming from a creative place? Were you physically making something the last time you felt joy: knitting a sweater, painting a picture, refinishing furniture, or writing a song. Whatever it was, try bringing life back to that old inspiration and see what happens. Then, gather the resources you need and start – one step at a time. You'll feel invigorated as you go.

If you are the type of person who is interested in learning about different cultures, this might be the perfect time to plan an extensive trip, to several cities within your country; or traveling abroad. Traveling might ignite that fire inside, once more. There are a number of ways to travel: solo, groups, exchange programs, expat associations, and the like. Anything is possible once you make up your mind that this is my objective. All you have to do is be courageous, research, plan, and connect. Your options are almost – limitless. This is where you can engage your interests, time and imagination to make it happen.

What if you're not the adventurous type and want to do something less-daring than traveling the world? Start small. The internet offers a world of vicarious experiences, right from the comfort of your own home. You can jot down what you learn in a notebook about places, people, DIY projects, conventions, festivals and so on, until you hit pay-dirt! Then, choose some activity and work towards making it happen. From there, reach out to others in various groups on social platforms to find like-minded people. Who knows, there may be a group that's already doing the same kinds of things you'd enjoy. So, go for it!

Contrary to the popular saying, "age is nothing, but a number," that's not totally true. So, when you start looking at new endeavors, consider your age, even if you're in excellent health. Once we hit that mid-life stage: 50+, we must accept the reality that we have limitations. For instance, I used to pride myself on how far I could walk, climb hills, etc. But, that was 30 years ago. The last time I climbed a mountain, Diamond Head, in Hawaii, back in 2013, I thought I was going to die! In fact, no one in our tour group explained to me that our "hike" consisted of climbing a mountain. Had they informed me, I would have opted to sit pool-side, sipping on a Mai Tai, instead!

If you're wondering how to kick start this new life, try visiting a favorite, or new craft shop, or a store that is decorated with items that evoke your imagination. Spending time just browsing, taking in the wonderful fragrances, and holding craft-pieces in your hands, may jumpstart your creativity and lead to a whole new adventure or discovery. In fact, Gretchen Rubin, author of books on happiness, says that "engaging your senses is a way to connect anew with the world and spark a little joy at the same time." Try listening to some music that makes you smile, maybe from an old Broadway show, like "Annie."

One of my favorite places used to be video game shops. I could play centipedes for hours. The shop was always brimming with other game-lovers. And, as we all engaged in our own little world of gaming, we created this bond of like-mindedness, which created a sense of community. I haven't visited a game shop in decades, but that's about to change. The thought of competing with space Martians, and kicking their butts, causes a surge of adrenalin to rise up in me; I can't wait to face off with them again! If you still find yourself struggling to know how to activate your creative side, take the advice of Scott Glassman, a noted psychologist. He advises "if you struggle to lighten up and have fun, ask yourself: *If I were a child right now what would I be doing?"*

Another great way to engage your mind is to move your body. I notice that whenever I'm stressed, getting up and moving my body, almost instantly, relieves the tension in both my mind and body. Establish an exercise routine. You could start exercising 10-15 minutes three times per day. If your daily routine is already hectic, be mindful about how you move. Use the stairs instead of the elevator, if you're healthy enough; walk a few times per week. Or, walk with co-workers at lunch.

If you don't work, or work from home, walk around your neighborhood. While you're at it, engage in some mindfulness activities, like bird-watching or deep-breathing for 5-10 minutes, while you walk. This mental-health break may even be better if you add a little soothing music, i.e. classical or nature sounds to the mix. The key is consistency.

Starting anew is harder said than done; so don't be afraid to get some help from a professional, clergy, or trusted family doctor. I know how much the right mental-health professional can be an anchor during those first few years when trying to come-to-terms with irreversible hardships and regrets. So, don't be a hero! Get some help until you feel steady enough to go it alone. Then, check in at least once per year with your trusted confidant. Trust me; you'll be glad you did. They'll help you decipher between reality and fantasy, which is one of your greatest struggles. Also, there are a variety of self-help groups online.

As you feel yourself shedding the painful scaffolding of the past, start thinking about what you want your future to look like. Ask yourself: is there one major change I need to make. For example, are you feeling restless? Should I explore making a move to another neighborhood, city, state or even country? If so, start investigating those feelings. Use a notebook or folder, so you can just start jotting down ideas that come to mind about the future. Would this new future require new skills? You could register for a few classes at the local community college, which oftentimes provide free life-long learning classes. What about tapping into some groups that may have similar interests? Since the pandemic, a number of groups have popped up. Check them out and see how you feel about becoming a member. Remember, you are engaging in a fact-finding mission, at this point and you want as many ideas as possible to cull from before making any final decisions. If after that time has passed, you still feel like a geographical move is what you need to feel free of the past, start planning places to visit. These places should be in line with your values as a person and provide the type of community you need to feel safe and included. Be open to meeting new and different people. What you needed ten or fifteen years ago may not be what will make you happy today. So, put on your explorer hat; just go with the flow and see what happens. Look at this period as the "question and answer" phase of your plan. The more questions you get affirmative answers to, the closer you may come to finding your new forever home. At the end of the year, if you are still indecisive, or decide moving isn't what you need, stay put. You can re-start this whole process over the next year. When the time is right to make a decision, you'll know, and make the right move.

These next suggestions are ones that I highly recommend for all of us. Take a **personality assessment** test, and **practice kindness**, (*order one of my: Choose to Be Kind t-shirts, at Beaconwear on Walmart*) to yourself and others. I know when you've been through hell and high-water, the last thing we usually think about is – others! After all, it was *others* that caused us so much pain. But, we must learn to separate those "others" from strangers and new friendships we may establish in the future. One way or another, we have to connect to people in order to be fully-alive. Thus, practice kindness. When you pass a stranger on the street, smile and say "Hello!" Or, if you're at the grocery store, strike up a conversation with another person while squeezing that cantaloupe. Ask someone how they make their spaghetti sauce, or what goes good with lamb chops? You never know where a simple discussion about recipes, could lead, a new friendship, or even a date (:

Forging into the future doesn't mean you need to change who you are; so remember to maintain certain boundaries. Or, before you know it, you could be reliving some nightmarish-type relationship(s) from the past. No still means no! Furthermore, let folks know that you may not be able to get right back to them. If you don't, it doesn't mean you're ignoring them; it just means you have some priorities that must be attended to first. However, let them know that you'll get back to them as soon as you can. Also, don't feel obligated to accept every invitation. Sure, it's great to be included, but only accept those dates that really align with your spirit. For example, if someone is throwing a charity event and you feel the need to give back; this would be one of those times to extend yourself, even if you'd rather stay at home watching old favorites, like the "Golden Girls." Helping those in need is inspirational!

If truth be told, past wounds are oh-so hard to heal. I know this for a fact; our best efforts may betray us, whereby we find ourselves repeating the same deeply-ingrained behavior patterns of the past. You'd be surprised to realize how hard it is to catch yourself acting badly. The reason, you can't. We're generally not able to act, and review the action at the same time. That's why it's only after we've said the wrong thing or approached someone in the wrong way, that we perceive how awful we behaved. But, then it's too late. At this point, we need to be open to getting help from a professional. There's no need to feel guilty, self-conscious or inadequate. The fact is we've been saddled with some emotional or psychological baggage that we can't dissolve on our own. For those of us who believe in a higher-power, spending more time in that space should be part of your healing process. If you don't, then seek out a professional experienced in trauma to help you navigate your way forward. Don't be surprised if you find yourself having to seek help again and again, before you get that breakthrough you need. Once the soul (i.e. the mind), is severely-compromised, it's a long-haul to getting back on the right road; but get back we must. So, promise yourself that you won't give up on you. If you do, who will be able to celebrate your victory? Remember, as you are healing, be gentle with yourself. You deserve as much compassion as do others. Also, be honest about your issues.

I spoke about *forgiveness* at the start of this discussion, but it is so important to being able to move forward, I wanted to make certain that my readers had a full-grasp of what forgiveness is, and the pivotal part it plays in the ability to move to a higher level of life.

It can't be emphasized enough that reconciling the very deep painful and stagnating feelings that un-forgiveness leaves in the pit of your soul, causes. The fact of the matter is, those of us who have been severely-traumatized also carry the burden of healing our own souls. That burden seems so unfair; in that the weight of such a burden can seem untenable as it is. Now, I/you have to forgive those who caused it? What a travesty of justice! Yes. I know. As they say: Life isn't fair; but, live, we must.

Thus, here is a more extensive overview of the act of forgiveness, along with some additional information you'll want to keep in mind: What it is; why it's important, and how you may navigate the process of forgiveness with a clear mind and light heart as you move forward.

Forgiving past hurts will look different depending on your specific set of circumstances, but in general it starts with a purposeful *intention and action* to extend forgiveness to another, or others, as the case may be. You must decide to let go of the resentment, anger or regret caused by the hurt. The pain you feel may remain, but letting go of the hatred will only benefit you.

As noted philosopher Carl Jung states, (in the Collected Works of Carl Jung, Vol 13),

"Facing the darkness in our lives takes courage, perseverance and self-discipline. First, we need to become aware of our suffering and false beliefs that hold us back from our authentic selves. This can be uncomfortable and scary because painful feelings that are buried will surface. We also might need to give up self-destructive behavior that has been our solace. Alternatively, we may need to forgive someone who has harmed us, or end a relationship. Whatever the outcome of our enlightenment, we have positively shifted our lives forever."

Let me unpack Carl Jung's quote. To know ourselves, we've got to "know ourselves." This means anything standing in the way of us exhibiting our "highest expression," must be faced and dealt with. Clearly, holding grudges, pain and resentment, from the past, will not allow us to express our highest good. Thus, living in bitterness does cause a deep-seated level of darkness to root in our souls, causing us to live a pseudo-life, not our best life.

Think of forgiving like unpacking a suitcase, after a long trip. In order to wash the dirt out of the clothes left after your trip, you must first, take them out of the suitcase (think of your soul as the suitcase); then sort them, and finally place them in piles, (prioritize your issues) according to color, fabric, and the like. Next, you've got to set the temperature (which of your issues are in need of more intense effort) of the washing machine and decide on the cycle (timeline for resolving these issues) you need to wash each pile of clothing. If you are going to be successful at forgiving someone, you will have to engage in a similar process. Just like some clothes will be harder to get clean, figure out which people will be harder to forgive. Use the appropriate temperature (i.e. your temper, or demeanor), when approaching them. And, decide on the best cycle to use. Will a quick rinse cycle work? Or, do you need a more carefully-planned wash? One person may only require a quick phone conversation; while another may require setting up a coffee date, to hash out all of the factors that led to your being harmed; and, plan what you want to say about how you feel. But, ultimately, the long or short of these interactions should end in forgiveness; hopefully, they'll be willing to fess-up as to their hurt feelings as well; and you both can leave your meeting feeling much lighter.

Forgiving frees not only your soul, but your mind. I don't have to tell you how awful carrying the burden of anger can become. It can color your entire life in a dark, dingy grey. You feel heavy, like you're carrying a heavy bag of junk around with you, that you just can't seem to put down. Eventually, something has to give, your anger or your health. According to the article, Healthy Living: Adult Health, by the Mayo Clinic:

"The act that hurt or offended you might always be with you. But working on forgiveness can lessen that act's grip on you. It can help free you from the control of the person who harmed you. Sometimes, forgiveness might even lead to feelings of understanding, empathy and compassion for the one who hurt you."

Have you ever had an experience whereby you found yourself having empathy for someone who wronged you? I have; and, it's powerful. Let me expound, just for a moment. There was this person I had a relationship with, when I was in my early-twenties. This person had some qualities that I admired; however, this person was very cruel, selfish, and self-centered, resulting in many years of agony. After our relationship ended, I suffered a great deal of emotional pain and financial hardship because of how the person treated me, including abandoning me when I was at one of the lowest points in my life. Somehow, I garnered enough strength to go on, but I was only a shell of my former self. The memories of the harsh treatment at that person's hands were never far away. Thus, I was operating at 50% at best; meaning I was basically treading water and going no-where fast. Eventually, I was able to find new meaning in life and forge a new future, in a new state. Still, the remnants of that horrible person, lingered; and, from time to time, something would happen that forced me to deal with the residual of being in relationship with that person. I felt those same old feelings return of anger, resentment, regret, loss, and hopelessness. Nevertheless, I was becoming stronger. I didn't let the scars left by that person dictate my future, anymore.

One day, about thirty years later, I heard that he'd died. At first, I felt relieved. The world seemed better with him being gone; but when I found out how he died, my feelings changed. Even though, he never apologized, or ever acknowledged that he had wronged me, I felt sorry for him. Suddenly, I was able to see him for who he really was – a self-loathing, weak, arrogant unforgiving, nobody, who always wanted to be somebody that he just didn't have the character, self-awareness or inner-love to become. I found myself stunned at these revelations. All of the years I'd allowed him to hold me hostage by my rage against him; a person who turned out not to have been worth the energy and emotions I expended, stunned me. I'd wasted years, decades, on what was nothing more than a lost cause anyway. Gosh, I felt like a fool; while at the same time, I felt free. I was finally free! But, why did this person have to die for me to see what was so evident. He was not up to my standards. We didn't share morals, values, outlook on life, what was important, and what wasn't. Had I only saw it then, I could have lived the previous three decades in bliss.

What I understand now is that childhood trauma prevents us from seeing ourselves for who we really are. Hence, we're vulnerable to users and others who are less than we deserve.

So, if you're feeling that you can never feel any empathy toward the person(s) who hurt you, think again. Just don't wait as long as I did, wasting 30 years in the process. See the person for who they are, good or bad. And, act accordingly.

How do you move toward forgiving someone? Make the decision to forgive. Then try the following:

- Realize the benefit of forgiveness and how it can improve your life: less anger, better mental health, etc.
- List the person(s) that you need to forgive and how doing so will bring about healing for you and them.
- Seek support via a group or therapy.
- Face up to your emotions and the harm you've endured because of these emotions: work, relationships, interests
- Decide to forgive the person(s) that caused you pain.

- Release the control and power those who hurt you have had on your life.
- Tell yourself it's really over.

Use empathy when thinking about the person that hurt you. Seeing the situation from the other person's point of view sometimes gives you a new perspective; and may lead to a better understanding of why they did what they did. This doesn't excuse what they did, but it will help to understand why they did what they did.

The goal in forgiveness is not necessarily to reconcile. There are many times when you never want to deal with the person – again! But, in order to go forth, you must release the grip that the pain they inflicted upon you has by forgiving the perpetrator of that pain. There's no other way to emotional healing and regeneration.

By the same token, if you are the one who needs forgiveness, be open if someone that you hurt reaches out to you. Maybe you have wanted to get this "monkey-off-your-back" too and their invitation may just be what you've been secretly waiting for; especially if you're the kind of person who can't admit that you're wrong. So, be prepared to humble yourself and accept that invitation.

If the person that hurt you refuses to resolve the issues, then forgive them anyway; release them from your heart, and wish them well. And, if they should change their mind, be receptive. It's always better to try to heal old wounds than to leave those festering until they cause real harm. Try visualizing that person in a more favorable way.

We can learn to forgive. According to Dr. Karen Swartz, M.D, of Johns Hopkins Hospital:

"Forgiveness is not just about saying the words. "It is an active process in which you make a conscious decision to let go of negative feelings whether the person deserves it or not. As you release the anger, resentment and hostility, you begin to feel empathy, compassion and sometimes even affection for the person who wronged you."

Dr. Swartz goes on to suggest using the following strategies in the process of learning to forgive:

Reflect and remember.

That includes the events themselves, and also how you reacted, how you felt, and how the anger and hurt have affected you since.

- Empathize with the other person.

For instance, if your spouse grew up in an alcoholic family, then “anger” when you have too many glasses of wine, might be more understandable, says Swartz.

Forgive deeply.

Forgiving may be enough to bring some healing. But one study found that people whose forgiveness came in part from understanding that *no one is perfect* were able to resume a normal relationship with the other person, even if that person never apologized. Those who only forgave in an effort to salvage the relationship wound up with a worse relationship.

Let go of expectations.

An apology may not change your relationship with the other person or elicit an apology from him/her. If you don't expect either, you won't be disappointed.

Decide to forgive.

Once you make that choice, seal it with an action. If you don't feel you can talk to the person who wronged you, write about your forgiveness in a journal or even talk about it to someone else in your life that you trust.

Forgive yourself.

The act of forgiving includes forgiving yourself. For instance, if your spouse had an affair, recognize that the affair is not a reflection of your worth, says Swartz

Now, that I've thoroughly-depressed you, let's talk about happier stuff. How about creating some fun ways to cope? This may sound crazy, but, what about creating a scream room? You could set it up where it's sound-proof to some degree, if you have neighbors, or other family members you don't want to disturb. Or, how does a punch-out room sound? You could fill it with punching bags, some other punch-able objects, like mannequins, stuffed animals, etc. Then, once-in-a-while, when you just have had it up to here, you can close yourself up in your special room, and have at it? Boy, how many relationships we might save, if we could contain our anger until we could let it out appropriately? Hey, you may even realize the other person was right all along; or, you may come up with a better approach to having that conversation next time. Either way, it's better to handle your frustration privately, than to unload on some unsuspecting bloke. Trust me, I know. Once the cat is out of the bag, you can't put it back.

There's a saying "Men don't cry;" but, that's a lie! I know it to be a truth that strong men do cry. Crying is very cathartic. I try to cry (though I'm a lady, so this is nothing unusual) at least once per week. It has a real calming effect, and it can even allow you to think more clearly, giving you the opportunity to concentrate on positive solutions, such as letting go of a situation that has simply run-its-course. So, don't be ashamed to let it all out once and a while. Consider those tears of joy!

You may have heard of this next idea. It's using affirmations to remind you of the truths or objectives you are aiming to reach. Use them as daily motivation.

We all are reaching for a balanced life, one where we feel content, included, and one in which we can express our true gifts. In many cases; however, there are those one or two behaviors, beliefs, or personality traits that keep interfering with us accomplishing the kind of life that would make us feel whole. You have the power to change!

Creating and reciting affirmations can help to re-program our thinking such that it eventually transforms our view of ourselves, others and the world. In order for affirmations to be effective, they must match the truth we want to attain, not the flawed self we are now. So, for instance, you may start with a few simple affirmations like the following:

- I AM Worthy (of – fill in the blank)
- I AM Loved or Loveable

- I Can Create an Atmosphere of Peace
- I Control What I Think and Feel, and Say

These statements should be recited at least three times per day. As you go about your daily routine, try to feel and behave in a manner that demonstrates your confessed affirmations. Of course, in the beginning of this process, you will have lapses; you'll behave in the pre-conditioned way you've learned all your life. That's okay. This is a learning process that can take years. Just be committed to the end-goal: mental, physical wellness, and a life worth living. As you get stronger at exhibiting these new more positive behaviors, you'll find your confidence is growing in parallel. The social *dis-ease* you once felt around strangers, will sub-side. You'll find yourself waiting to form an opinion of people until you have all the facts; which may take several encounters with them before you really know what kind of person with whom you're dealing. That's what you want – control. When we can control our responses (i.e. our emotional responses), we give ourselves an advantage. Remember, that first impression is a lasting one. And, as I said before, once the cat (the wrong words, etc.) is out-of-the-bag, you can't put it back. So, control is big when it comes to dealing with others. We want to repair the damaged filters in our mind.

Knowing what you want to accomplish in the future, intellectually, is important; but being able to visualize it is even more powerful. Visualization uses your natural creative instincts to think through your goals and make a plan for the future.

Here's a brief overview of how to create a vision board that encompasses the new life you want to build.

- Start by thinking about what's important to you as a person, a citizen of the world, a worker or business owner, etc. This would include things such as your values, morals, religious beliefs, and so on. Aligning your goals with who you are as a person can be a powerful motivator in achieving your goals. If this exercise seems difficult to you, start with asking yourself some questions, including:

- What do I want to be? What's important to me? Where do I see myself in 5, 10, or 15 years? What are some first steps I can take to move closer to my objectives? Where do I want to live? What gives me meaning? How can I turn my skills into a job?

- Hash-out each of the questions you've identified above by delving deeper into each and writing up a one-page summary for each question. For example:

- Who am I? That's a potentially loaded question, but the most important one. You may want to get some help with this one. Taking a personality quiz or a whole slate of personality assessments would be a great help in hashing the answers out on this question.

- Use imagery (i.e. vision board, mind map) to help you get a visual of who you are, like old photos from trips you've taken, special tokens from college, birthday parties, church events, and other times when you felt happy. Tape all these mementoes into a notebook or folder, and add whatever decorations you want that enhances these memorable events in your life.

- Set priorities. It's one thing to want something; but it's a totally different thing to achieve that objective. Focus your plan on the most feasible goals first. Once you've achieved that one, go on to the next most possible goal. You should set a time limit for each goal. One to three years for each goal is sufficient for realistic goals. It's, okay to re-set priorities as necessary.

- Organize your vision board to reflect the highest priorities to the lowest. Create a visual representation of these priorities. This can be the really fun part of your vision board. Use images that elicit joy, fun, curiosity, adventure, and hope. For example, you could use an image of a mountain. Place images that represent your highest goal at the very top. Say, you want to complete your certification as a ski instructor. You can cut out a picture of skis, skier, or a ski lift, and glue it to the top of the mountain. Next, say you want to write a children's book, glue an image of a children's book on the next lowest level of the mountain. When you've completed this visual representation of your vision board, you'll have a beautiful illustration of what your goals are and how you see your life in the future. This visual will be a constant reminder of where you're headed; and along with the written portion of your vision board, the steps/actions you're going to employ to achieve these goals.

- Divide your vision board up into sections

  - Career
  - Travel
  - Health
  - Money
  - Personal life
  - Other relationships

Create a vision board for all of these goals, simultaneously, or create one for each goal, individually, can act as a clear-guide to decision-making in your life.

To make this creative process more fun, invite a few friends, co-workers, or others to join you in a "Vision Board" party, outing, or group. This way, you guys can bounce ideas off of each other. And, if one of your goals is to travel, voila! You'll have a whole group to invite on your adventure. Not, to mention, all of you are already in the "seeking mode." So, it's a good bet that one or more would be in for a good excursion, rather local, or beyond. In fact, I think this is such a good idea, bringing people together to create their vision boards for their future, I'm recommending it as a "must" engagement for anyone who is ready to tap into their inner-child and rediscover their true essence.

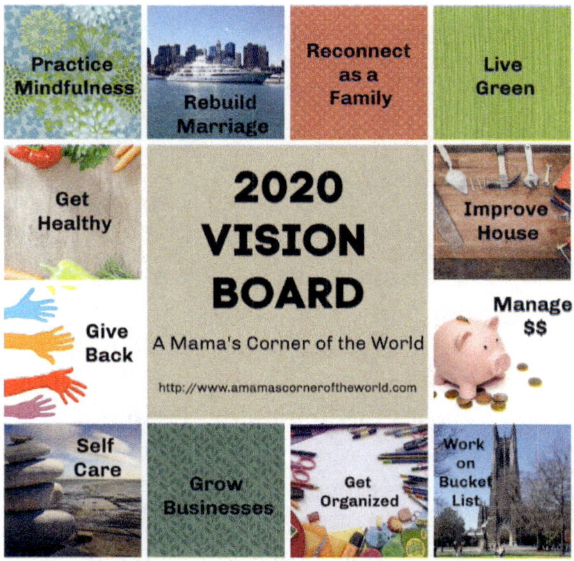

This is a very well-done vision board that clearly separates life into twelve sections focused on what's important in this person's life. I think this example would make a great one to mimic as you're planning your own vision board. It covers all the most important aspects of life – to consider.

Another very powerful practice is meditation. This process takes a myriad of forms. You can find a number of types of meditation on the internet, but I would suggest something simple. For example, if you suffer from anxiety, search for meditations that are designed to lower anxiety levels. Start slow and build as you become more knowledgeable. The key is to be consistent. If you can find ten to fifteen minutes a day (twice per day), to engage in this centering exercise, you may experience a dramatic shift in the level of anxiety you feel.

Closely-related to meditation is something referred to as mindfulness. In the hectic, and increasingly complex world we live, many of us, are operating on autopilot. Sometimes, we can’t tell our head from our feet. That’s a problem. Slowing down and becoming aware of what we're doing, feeling and thinking, in the moment, is central to having a healthier mind and body. Mindfulness involves stopping and taking an assessment of ourselves. It may involve just sitting for five minutes and asking ourselves: How am I feeling, right now? Did I eat a proper meal today? What were my goals for today; did I accomplish them? Am I dealing with any stress? If so, what am I doing to handle it for the best outcome? Do I need help to handle my issues? What resources should I consult?

Asking yourself questions about your state of mind will go a long way to helping you focus on what's most important to you in the moment. It will also help you determine next steps that need to be taken to remedy issues that are urgent or that you uncover during this process. However you go about your mindfulness process, don't be afraid to seek help if things seem a little too complicated.

The key to our entire future is our mental and physical well-being. Thus, it has to be at the very top of our list when it comes to improving our life experience. All of the ideas I've shared up to now, feed into this next one.

You need to love yourself before you can truly love anyone else.

This should be easy, but we all know it can be the hardest thing we ever do. Think of self-care like car care. If you keep your car well-maintained, it runs like a charm; but ignore it for a couple years, and you may end up with a huge repair bill. Such is the case with self-care. Our body is like our car frame. It houses a lot of important stuff that needs periodic servicing to run effectively. Inside our frame is our vital organs, blood (i.e. fuel in our car), bone structure, brain, etc. These parts all combine to make up our human car. And, unlike a metal car, we can't replace most of it, albeit a few parts can be replaced. But, by the time our human car needs parts replaced, we're in bad shape. I'm all for keeping my original parts in good running-order, instead of the serious and sometimes very dangerous process of replacing these parts. But, to do that, you've got to be on top of your game! Just like you take care of your house, car, clothes, and other inanimate objects, you've got to put a laser-focus on our health. To do this, especially if you're not accustomed to paying attention to your health, I'd suggest starting a health journal. What do I mean? If you can see it, you can change it.

When you were in middle, high school or college, you had to keep a notebook with all your assignments, and the test scores you received so that you could look back over your performance and gage how well you'd done. Those reports helped you prepare for the final. Health Journals can help you keep track of how well you've done month-to-month; year-to-year; or week to week. In fact, I think a great idea would be to combine your health journal with your mindfulness work. This way, you could see how you're doing in terms of managing your stress, tasks, and your health simultaneously. Approaching self-care in this manner may save time and give you a more comprehensive view of how you're doing overall, in the areas of health and life management. There are a number of ways you could approach combing mindfulness, and self-care. Using a notebook with pockets, you could keep evidence of special milestones in the pockets. Say, after practicing these healthy habits over two months, you notice how much better you feel when leading a discussion at work. Or, how much more calm you felt socially when meeting people for the first time. As a pat on the back, you could buy yourself a nice greeting card, which celebrates these accomplishments. Or, you could buy yourself a CD/DVD of your favorite artist and play it whenever you think of how far you've come on your journey to self-improvement. You could buy some tickets to see your favorite group in person. Staple the tickets to the front of your notebook, as a reminder of what you'll get if you stay-the-course. Hey, why not write several possibilities on scratch paper; then, shake up the bag and pull one out? Make choosing how to celebrate yourself a surprise! The possibilities are endless. Treat yourself just like you do others when they accomplish a goal. Be your own "cheer leader!"

Finally, don't forget to infuse some creativity (a big theme of mine) into your self-improvement journey. This may be the perfect time for you to revisit that scrap-booking project you abandoned five years ago. Or, remember how you used to love visiting vintage yard sales, why not start that hobby again? I know from personal experience how motivating being in the midst of a creative endeavor can be. It literally feeds my soul. It may do the same for you. So, allow your imagination to roam until that long-lost, once-loved, activity of old resurfaces in your mind. Then, grab-it-by-the-horns, and let it take you on a ride to your inner-child that may just last a lifetime. Bon Voyage!

I want to revisit what the experts say when it comes to raising our emotional frequency: Positive frequencies improve happiness; and, the ideas that lead to healthier mindsets, both of which determine our destiny.

To review, too much cortisol and/or adrenalin is the villain. If you find yourself pulling out your hair when that co-worker used your coffee cup once too many times, without asking, that's cortisol on steroids (pun intended; because cortisol is a steroid). There are many other examples of your cortisol/adrenalin levels going on tilt, like when someone cuts you off on the road, (could result in road rage); a rude person cuts in front of you at the theatre, or a person standing right on top of you in the check-out line at the grocery store, trying to force you to hurry up and finish your purchase so they can check out. These inappropriate behaviors (theirs and potentially your response) are usually caused by an overdose of cortisol/adrenalin – the stress hormones. These two hormones are so powerful that reams of literature, treatments, and therapies have been compiled to help us manage and recalibrate the levels of these hormones within our neurological system. Adjusting these stress-response hormones are literally a *matter of life and death*.

Think of how many stories you've watched on the evening news, involving people who did something so terrible, that you said, out loud, to yourself, "He/She is nuts!" Or, "They must be crazy to have done that!" Well, that's how powerful unregulated adrenalin/cortisol can become – deadly. So, we want to pay close attention to our responses; especially, when under stress. Ask yourself: Did I respond normally? If the answer is no, you need to seriously think about getting some professional help. The exposure to increased levels of cortisol and adrenalin, over long periods of time, can literally cause brain damage. And, once the brain is damaged, sorry to say, it can't be repaired back to the pre-damaged state. It can only be managed. So, when you hear or read about people having chronic depression, PTSD, and the like, those are examples of permanent brain damage. The moral to the story: responding in a temperate manner to some annoyances can save more than your job, or relationship. It might just save your brain health; without which, your life will only be an exercise in surviving one crisis after another. According to Everlywell, (2023), an online blog:

"Cortisol and adrenaline are closely linked, and they play an intrinsic role in your overall health. Managing stress and learning how to reduce stress hormones, by keeping cortisol and adrenaline levels down, is essential to maintaining a healthy quality of life."

There's a resource, where you can find a list of foods that help with reducing stress, in the *resources* section at the back of this book.

The key to feeling better about yourself and your life is to raise your frequency or vibration from low (negative emotions) to high (positive emotions). For instance, when you're happy, you feel a sense of accomplishment or joy. Those feelings are rated as being high-frequency or vibration feelings; whereas sadness is rated lower on the frequency/vibration chart. And, though there is no definitive data to prove the aforementioned, two experts in the area of the subject, introduced the *emotional frequency chart*. They are Dr. David R. Hawkins and Abraham Hicks, both have conducted extensive research on how our emotions vibrate depending on if they're positive vs negative. In short, their research show positive emotions radiate high frequencies or vibrations; and negative emotions do the opposite. Based on the research that these two experts conducted, a chart called, the "Emotional Frequency Chart" was created. It rates emotions on a vibrational scale. Emotions are given a frequency rating, and those, such as joy, love, passion, receive a higher frequency rating than sadness, shame, or anger. Though not scientific, it makes sense that positive emotions would generate a higher frequency than negative. To help people move up in the emotional frequency rating, there are 7 recommendations that came out of Dr. Hawkins, and Mr. Hicks' research; and you can use them in your life, if you wish, to help raise your emotional frequency ratings. The following chart comes from an article by Ryan Kane, on the mindfulness website, dated October 3, 2023. You may refer back to that reference for further information.

7 steps to raise your frequency

1. Set the right expectations. Jumping straight from shame to joy isn't a realistic path, and it won't feel authentic.

2. Do high vibrational activities like exercise, meditation, journaling, and being in nature.

3. Be around high vibrational people. The people you're around are highly influential to your mood and state of being.

4. Practice gratitude. Start practicing daily to build your gratitude muscle.

5. Help others. When you're not sure how to move yourself into a higher vibrational state, it always pays to think about what you car do for others.

6. Make time to play. Figure out what your inner child wants and make more time for playful activities.

7. Understand that progress isn't linear. You'll still have good and bad days.

The process described above will be easy for some and scary for others. It's difficult to change how you think and act overnight. As you put these steps into action, accept that frustration is a part of the practice of elevating your positive frequency levels. Using your affirmations, when you feel frustrated, or when you want to quit, will be a big help here. Affirmations including:

- I AM GROWING WITH EVERY POSITIVE CHANGE I MAKE
- I WILL NOT ALLOW FEAR TO HAVE THE FINAL SAY.
- I'M CLOSER TO A BETTER TOMORROW

THAN I WAS

YESTERDAY

Will go a long way to push you past the point where you want to give up. Make a decision, that changing your way of responding to stressful situations, from negative to more positive, is not an option! And, if you should fall short, as we all do, forgive yourself. Remember, part of the entire process of being successful at employing any of the strategies in this book, is the ability to *forgive* – yourself and others. To give you another tool in your process of learning how to forgive, use the following reconciliation diagram. Practice the following steps with a friend, family member, or other willing participant.

THE PROCESS OF FORGIVING

The following chart uses the word, RESOLVE, to provide steps in the process of reconciliation. It's easy to follow, and uses a commonsense approach to reaching some level of resolution to conflict. Practicing these steps will help you develop your conflict resolution skills.

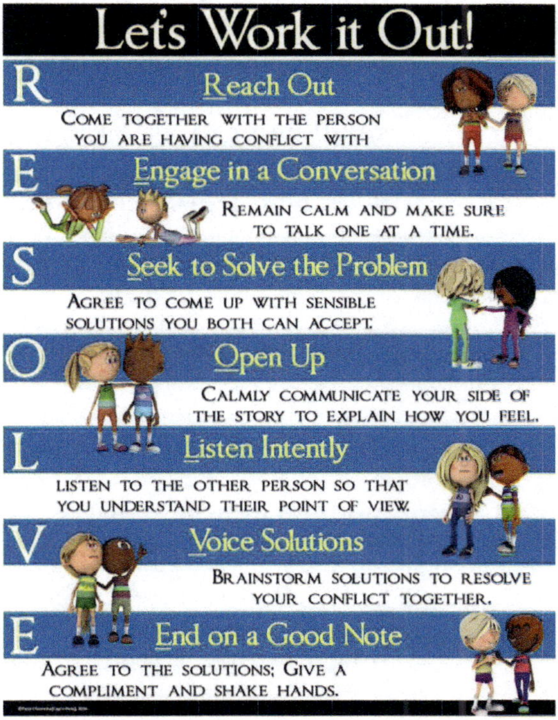
Let's Work it Out!
R
Reach Out
COME TOGETHER WITH THE PERSON YOU ARE HAVING CONFLICT WITH
E
Engage in a Conversation
REMAIN CALM AND MAKE SURE TO TALK ONE AT A TIME.
S
Seek to Solve the Problem
AGREE TO COME UP WITH SENSIBLE SOLUTIONS YOU BOTH CAN ACCEPT.
O
Open Up
CALMLY COMMUNICATE YOUR SIDE OF THE STORY TO EXPLAIN HOW YOU FEEL.
L
Listen Intently
LISTEN TO THE OTHER PERSON SO THAT YOU UNDERSTAND THEIR POINT OF VIEW.
V
Voice Solutions
BRAINSTORM SOLUTIONS TO RESOLVE YOUR CONFLICT TOGETHER.
E
End on a Good Note
AGREE TO THE SOLUTIONS; GIVE A COMPLIMENT AND SHAKE HANDS.

These simple yet powerful conflict resolutions steps can make a huge difference in how you approach your relationships. Keep them in a small notepad, or on your phone. Then, when you feel like you're falling into a slump, pull them out and implement whichever one(s) that seem feasible.

Relationships, unfortunately, are unavoidable; they make up at least 50% of our lives. We have family relationships, friend relationships, neighbor relationships, work relationships, and I could go on and on.

Therefore, seriously thinking about how to raise your emotional vibrations and developing greater self-control, in an ever-changing world, is worth the effort. Of course, you could become a hermit (I've tried), but even still, you're going to have to come in contact with people, even if just at the local grocery store or post office. There's no way to control who and when we interact with other people, so we just have to face facts. We need to be better at interpersonal communications.

It may seem like I'm harping on stuff you feel you already know; but take it from someone who has suffered a lifetime of unnecessary hardships, because of low emotional frequency issues. Things can go south, fast, when dealing with people; and before you know it, you could be looking for a new job or a new spouse; when if you'd only kept your cool, things could have worked out more-smoothly. This is not to say you weren't thinking of making those changes anyway; but, why go through excess drama, heartache, financial distress, or worse, because you didn't know how to control yourself? There's a better way; and, I know the saying, "You can't teach an old dog, new tricks." But, after spending untold hours in some court(s), or shelling out extra money for moving expenses, or (heaven forbid), having to move back in with the folks, you'll have a change of attitude and approach to life.

Now, most of us older folks may have learned these things the hard way; but, you (if you're under 40) can be a *beacon* of sorts, to the younger generation. They haven't learned half of what we forgot about life. So, make sure you load up on copies of this book to give as gifts to teens, young adults, or older adults, who refuse to grow up. They'll thank you for it later, when they've "*dodged a bullet*" that could have cost them – big time!

Speaking of teaching old dogs new tricks, it helps to have as many strategies as possible when you find yourself stressed and not feeling very blessed. Hold fast to the following suggestions, and use them to bring you back from the brink, when life seems to be tilting toward disaster.

- Find a sacred place or space that calms your nerves and just dwell there for an hour. Have a cup of tea, coffee, or whatever your favorite (non-alcoholic) beverage is and let it sooth your soul. Think on better times.
- Avoid fatalistic thinking (my Achilles heel). In fact, try thinking of that last time

you felt joy or contentment and focus on that. Doing so, will help you realize: This too shall pass.

- Take out a sheet of paper (or a napkin, if that's what's available) and start jotting down words that represent what you want to accomplish in this moment. For instance, if you're dealing with a financial emergency, you might write down: yard sale, refinance, reconsolidate, etc. These words will begin to generate other ideas in your mind related to resolving the financial difficulties you're facing.

- Think of a bible verse that will anchor you when you start feeling like things are just too hard for you to deal with. For example, "I can do all things through Christ, which strengthened me," (Philippians, 4:13). You'll find your strength coming back and you'll be able to fight on and stand in this time of trouble. Scripture is a powerful ally.

- Listen to music, whatever the genre, as long as it lifts your spirit, is good. Many solutions came to me while I was listening to my favorite gospel artist.
- Get into nature. Walking in a park, where there are a lot of trees; and especially, a body of water, like a creek, can have a magical effect on the spirit of a person; before you

know it, an idea that you couldn't ever have imagined, pops up in your mind; and, suddenly, your problem is resolved.

- Be your own best friend. It can be very hard to overcome challenges alone; but, sometimes all we have is ourselves. Does that mean you should cave when you come under opposition? Heck no! What it means is that you have to fight harder, stay positive about you, and if possible garner support from others as you move toward solving the problem that you face. But, by no means give up. Tell yourself, like, Gloria Gaynor, "I will survive!"

- Be gentle and kind to yourself.

Like the suggestion above, be your own best friend; and don't be too hard on yourself when you lose it. We're all just fragile human beings. So, remember everybody is struggling. You are not alone in this fight.

- Let Google be your personal assistant. Can't afford an attorney? No worries. Whatever the issue, you can begin to become more informed by using this awesome search engine. Whether consumer laws, or the best meditation videos for depression, Google can give you a running start to the information you need. I never leave home without it(:

- Read personal narratives of people who overcame seeming insurmountable odds. (Google can help you there, too). The library holds a treasure trove of resources. Visit a library, you may re-discover that love for reading you once had.
- Date yourself. I do this all the time. At least once a week, I take myself somewhere that makes me feel special. Places like a craft store where I

can browse through DIY books. Or, a large café/bookstore, where I'll have a cup of hot chocolate, while perusing Life Magazine, or some such (: And, if I have a few extra dollars, I'll take in a new release at a movie theatre. You'd be surprised what a couple hours of bliss can do for your spirit.

- Declutter. This is worth reiterating, if I've already mentioned it; because, there's nothing so freeing as getting rid of the junk taking up space in your home. This is especially true, if you live in a smaller abode, like an apartment.

- Workout. I said this before, but I'm repeating it here, so you'll know how (very) important this is; and, how hard it is when you're feeling blue. Well, one of the most effective things against this stress build up, is to "Move that Body!" Yeah! Get up off the floor, couch, bed, or from wherever you're having your pity party;

and let the music play, as you dance the night away. Oh, wait. I think that line comes from a song (: But, you get my meaning. Right? So, boogie, do jump-in-jacks, stretch, or plain old dance until the vibrations become lighter and more positive. Then, go after the problem you're facing with a renewed spirit and determination to slay that dragon and regain control of your life.

- Laugh! Now, it's easier said than done; especially

when you're dealing with a life-challenging situation; but, if there's anything you can do, i.e. an outing at a local comedy event, watch re-runs of your favorite 90's comedy, rent a video of some blockbuster movie that featured the funniest comics of our time. Or, read the funnies in the local newspaper. Do it; because laughter boost happy hormones, like oxytocin, dopamine and serotonin, which are naturally occurring chemicals that help to regulate our mood.

- Join group therapy. Dealing with problems becomes easier if you can talk about it. The best people to talk to; however, about issues you're dealing with, are others dealing with the same or similar issues. Check your local community website for group counseling opportunities. Or, look up the American Psychological Association for references. There is no shame in reaching out for help; in fact, it's a sign of self-awareness and strength.

- Volunteer. You may be thinking, "The last thing I'd want to do is be around strangers when I'm going through hell!" But, getting out of your shell and seeing up-close what some of your neighbors are dealing with may be *just what the doctor ordered* to get you out of your slump. So, contact the local senior citizen center, Boys

& Girls club or church, and lend a hand. It will not only be much appreciated by the organization, but it'll help you out much more than you know. Just being able to forget your troubles for a while can work wonders for your mood, attitude, and outlook on the future. So, find someone to help, and see how much your mood improves.

The objective in this section is: Moving Forward. And, as you have seen, it takes a whole lot of assessing, planning, and action to change the old tapes running in your head; which is necessary to overcome the pain of the past and realize a potential better tomorrow. Here, you're playing the long game. Fix your mind to understand that "change" is the hardest thing you'll ever do. This is because, psychologically-speaking, by the time we're five years old our basic personality is set. The problem is, for many of us, the set was misconfigured, i.e. childhood trauma. As a result, many of us start out light waves behind those children who are nurtured with love, acceptance (there's that word again), and respect, verses just being tolerated. In essence, if you've been taught that you're bad, not accepted, not valuable, you will grow up with "low-self-esteem; thus, you are always the odd-man out. Can you recall your middle school experience, where there were certain people always selected to be a part of a team, or to sit next to at lunch. And, you wished that were you? Well, the difference between that person and us is that they were taught that they are valuable, loved and accepted, in childhood. We, on the other hand, must learn to love ourselves. Nevertheless, we deserve to feel loved, even if it's just our own.

To reiterate, the foundation of all of the above is forgiveness. Following, are four examples to show you how powerful forgiveness can be on your way to a better life.

The Widower

It's easy to say you're a Christian, but when tragedy hits, you have to put your money (or your faith), where your mouth is. That was the case for a young husband, father, and *pastor*, on a fateful day back in October of 2006.

Firefighter, Matt Swatzell, 20, was driving home after a 24 hour shift. He hadn't slept for quite some time, and was fatigued as he tried to make it to his residence. He fell asleep at the wheel, and his life would be changed forever. The man's life, who was the husband to the women driving the vehicle Swatzell hit, would also be changed forever. You see, Erik Fitzgerald's wife, June was driving that car and she had her 19 month old daughter, Faith (ironically) with her sitting in the rear of the vehicle. Fortunately, Faith survived, but her mother, June, who was pregnant with their second child, did not; neither did the unborn child.

Erik Fitzgerald was devastated, obviously, but instead of seeking revenge via the court system, which would have resulted in a long jail sentence for Swatzell, he was inspired to forgive. It took about two years for the judicial system to conclude the proceedings regarding Swatzell's matter, but before the sentencing could be finalized, Erik, the grieving spouse, knew he had to forgive his wife's killer. He told the judge at sentencing, that he did not want another life to be lost in this unfortunate tragedy. So, he requested leniency for Swatzell. The judge honored Fitzgerald's request.

Swatzell was sentenced to community service and paid a fine.

As a Christian and a pastor, Erik had studied the Holy Bible, and learned about the power of forgiveness. So, he sought Swatzell out, and told him he felt there was a reason he should be in his life; also, that he wanted to extend forgiveness to him. Somehow Erik Fitzgerald perceived that there was a greater purpose to the accident that took his wife and unborn child's life; and, forgiving the man who'd caused him so much loss was the key to this greater good. He knew that Faith was an action, not just a belief to be spoken of, but never acted upon.

The two men forged a friendship of sorts. They met for coffee, and/or lunch every couple of weeks; and eventually became genuine friends. Erik helped Swatzell, who was filled with deep guilt about the accident, to heal. That's where Erik's sincere forgiveness and support came into play. He knew that if he didn't help Swatzell overcome his guilt, another life would be lost. Erik embraced Swatzell as a brother-in-

Christ, and forgave him. As a result, Swatzell was able to overcome his guilt, and became a father and husband himself.

Erik Fitzgerald demonstrated the Christian principle that "we must forgive as we've been forgiven" by Christ. And, that is what we all must learn.

Mother's Love

Mary Johnson went from hating the youngster who killed her 20 year old (only) son, Laramiun Byrd, to calling him "son." What caused this unlikely transformation? Here's Mary's story.

It 1993, Mary was a mother who was trying to raise a son, alone, which is difficult enough, especially in a disadvantage community, where graduation rates are low, and the struggle to survive a constant companion. Laramiun was a dropout; and by the time of his death he hadn't finished high school. Statistics show that teens that don't finish high school are twice as likely as those who have completed high school to find themselves involved with the criminal justice system, on some level; whether as a victim or a victimizer. Unfortunately, Laramiun became the former. He was at the wrong place, at the wrong time; he didn't perceive the potential danger he was in when he encountered Oshea Israel. Perhaps, Laramiun thought because Oshea (he was 16 at the time of the incident) looked or seemed younger than him, he could step to him with no problem; but it turned out that would not be the case. Oshea was capable of great violence.

The facts of the story seemed to bear out that both teens were troubled. Oshea Israel was another troubled-teen; but was much more dangerous than the average troubled-teen. He apparently had a different kind of mindset: kill or be killed; because on the day he crossed paths with Laramiun, he was packing (carrying a gun), and was prepared to use it.

Two teens meeting at a party should be just another fun night; but the night Laramiun and Oshea crossed paths, was anything but fun. It turned deadly. The two got into some kind of argument, and a fight ensued. Unlike in the old days, when squabbles between young adults, were settled by fist-a-cups, guns are the equalizer of choice, today. And, unfortunately, when guns are involved, the result is often – deadly. When the smoke cleared, Laramiun, just 20 years old at the time, with his whole life ahead of him was dead. Whether he died at the scene, or at the hospital, really doesn't matter, his life came to a tragic end in the year of 1993.

To lose a son, tragically, is more than a mother can be expected to bare; but Mary Johnson, was not satisfied with expressing her rage or venting her grief amongst friends, family or other sympathetic people. No. She needed more! She wanted to know, "Why?" The pain in her heart fueled this need to speak to her son's killer and get the answers she needed, so that maybe one day she could find peace. As it turned out, Mary got more than she bargained for, when she finally spoke face-to-face with Oshea Israel. It took twelve years for this face-to-face meeting to occur; because Oshea had refused to meet with Miss Johnson, 11 years earlier, when she requested to meet with him to discuss his actions leading to her son's death. But, as the years rolled by, Oshea matured, and agreed to meet with his victim's mother, Mary Johnson.

The meeting between Mary Johnson and Oshea Israel occurred at

Stillwater Prison for Men, in Bayport, MN, in March 2005. Miss Johnson was curious to see if Oshea was still the same anger-filled, violent boy she remembered from the court hearings. To her surprise, he was not. Oshea, now 28 had mellowed, reflected on his pass and was ready to admit he was wrong for his actions that took Mary's son's life.

Mary told Oshea that she thought they should get to know one another; because he took the life of someone he didn't know. Nor did he know her, or she him. He agreed. They had a long talk that led to repentance on the part of Oshea and forgiveness on the part of Mary Johnson. In fact, this meeting turned out to be necessary for her healing. As she was about to leave this meeting with her son's killer, now a man, remorseful for his actions, she just broke down in tears. Oshea, having caused her enough pain, caught her in his arms; because he said, "He couldn't let her hit the floor." That hug freed Mary from over a decade of agony. She has since passed, but she is at peace.

Brotherly-Love Lost and Found

In 1962, Belgium relinquished control it held over African territory, resulting in two new countries, Rwanda and Burundi, being formed. Between 1962 and 1994, a number of violent clashes occurred between the Hutus and Tutsis; all of this was leading up to the genocide of 1994, (Britannica Encyclopedia).

Rwanda, an African nation, in Central/Eastern Africa, was under colonialist rule (by the British and Belgium), from roughly 1894-1994. After Belgium turned over control of Rwanda back to its people, a struggle ensued between the former aristocratic (deemed by Belgium to be better because they were light-skinned-mixed Africans), Tutsis, and the Hutus, (the darker-skin, and less valued by the white rulers, during the time of their captivity). This fight became bloody, as the Hutus sought revenge on the Tutsis for having not only been favored by their former white rulers, but for mistreating them, due to their less-than-favored status. It wasn't long before outright genocide was taking place. At the end of the fighting, over one million (mostly Tutsis) Rwandans were dead – due to the brutal fight for power.

Ten years after the 1994 Rwandan Genocide had ended, and to help the Rwandan people to forge reconciliation with their brothers and sisters, two non-profits in the country began offering classes to teach the people how to ask for forgiveness, and to pardon the ones who committed atrocities against them and their families. And, the president, Kagame, of the country at the time, also agreed to free any perpetrators of the genocidal acts, if they completed the program successfully, asked for forgiveness, and was pardoned by their victims. Many prisoners took the president up on his offer.

The reconciliation program was hugely- successful, despite the deep-seated pain, loss and anger the victims (the Tutsis) experienced at the hands of their fellow Rwandans (the Hutus), they all realized they had little choice if they wanted to move forward. As one of the survivors of the 1994 Rwandan Genocide, learned via the program,

''It is not fair to avenge your beloved one. It took time, but in the end we realized that we are all Rwandans. The genocide was due to bad governance that set neighbors, brothers, and sisters against one another. Now, you accept and you forgive. The person you have forgiven becomes a good neighbor. One feels peaceful and thinks well of the future."

-Cesarie Mukabutera, survivor, 1994 Genocide in Rwanda-

The reconciliation project that was started to help Rwandans recover from the genocide they endured has been chronicled in pictures and is available for viewing at Hague, The Netherlands.

This poignant example of people finding it in their best interests to forgive is no-doubt, one of the most extreme; but one of the most powerful. If the Rwandan people can forgive the absolutely most heinous acts of violence against themselves, and love ones, we who have never had to endure such unthinkable tragedy surely must learn to forgive as well.

The Greatest Love of All

And, for my last example, I would be remiss, if I neglected to speak about our *Lord and Savior, Jesus Christ*. Born in a manger; because there was no room for him at the Inn, comes the greatest love of all! Yes, the architect of creation, who came spreading love and forgiveness to all human kind, if you dare only to *believe in him and follow his commandments*.

Jesus Christ, the author and finisher of my (and your) life, is the epitome of the very idea of forgiveness. Over his thirty-three years on Earth, Jesus healed, forgave and saved many, like the lame man. This man had been sitting at the Sheep Gate Bethesda (the gate beautiful), for thirty-eight years, unable to make it to the pool of healing, because "no man would help me," he said to Jesus. This Gate had five porches. Here, lay many sick people, lame, paralyzed and, blind, waiting for the water to begin to swirl. (An angel would come down into the pool, at a certain time each day, and stir up the waters; and that meant someone would have the opportunity to be healed.) However, only the first person who stepped into the pool would have their ailment(s), healed. The lame man couldn't walk, so he had no way of getting to the pool, when the water stirred, let alone get there first. So, there he lay, with no hope; as everyone at the pool was sick and in need of healing. This was an "every man for himself situation."

Jesus and his disciples were on their way to a *feast of the Jews* in Jerusalem, and happened upon this scene at the Gate Beautiful, when he spotted the lame man. Jesus, knowing that the lame man had been in this case a long time, asked him, "Do you want to be healed?" Now, the man, not knowing this was Jesus, who asked the question, responded, "I have no man to help me get to the pool. As I am coming, another steps before me and gets into the pool." Notice, the man tells Jesus all his woes, how there's always some obstacle to him getting what he wants done. And, although he did perceive that Jesus was a man of stature, because he referred to him, as "Sir," he didn't perceive that this man, who was asking him about his *condition*, might have a solution to his problem; after all, he'd been there thirty-eight years, and no one else had helped him. Yet, he just bemoaned to Jesus about his *condition*, he was still in after all these years. Then, Jesus, realizing the man was not only lame, but blind (my interpretation), said to the man, "Rise, take up your bed (all your troubles, complaints, and concerns), and walk." And, instantly, the lame man, walked! What he couldn't do in thirty-eight years, the Power of God, through Jesus, was accomplished – in an instant. Praise the Lord!

The example of Jesus healing the lame man is just one of many. If you choose to read the Holy Bible, you'll learn of those. But, the greatest love God ever showed was when he sent Jesus to the Cross as a sacrifice for our sins. He died that we may live. You see, it took a spotless, guiltless, sacrifice to make up for the sins of humanity. In Jesus' sacrifice, all our sins are forgiven. And, that's the greatest love of all! But, don't be like the lame man – perceive! If the spirit moves you, receive Jesus into your heart and be restored and healed. To God is the Glory! In Jesus name, Amen and Amen!

You may learn more about Jesus, if you so choose, by reading the Holy Bible – KJV

Afterword

As we come to the end of this first part of our journey within, I'll leave you with a few thoughts.

Human beings tend to drift through life as though hypnotized, unaware of the beauty and possibilities that surround us. The reasons for this are many, but usually have to do with the need to be conformed to the systems of life: family dynamics; expectations between friends, spouses, or community; work requirements, or religious beliefs. While all of these formalities are necessary for societies to run smoothly, they can also be stifling, leading to mental distress and in severe cases, mental illness. It's safe to say, the later has become the norm. However, nature is our greatest healer; thus we always have the opportunity to renew, restore, and start anew. All we need to do is pay attention; and miracles of shifting perspectives may result in a life more worth living. That's what noticing a little frog did for me.

Namaste

About Author

Renā Johnson is a highly-skilled educator and spiritually-lead healer. She uplifts and empowers her readers and those she meets by reminding them that their past mistakes, family dysfunctions, or failures, do not define the totality of who they are now. And, who you are now is who you must embrace. That may take some help; but reading this book and following the suggestions herein is a start.

Over Renā's 25 years in the field of education, she observed how the impact of a student's self-awareness impacted their behavior. It became clear to her that those students who had loving caregivers, who accepted and supported them, fared far-better than those students who didn't. So, what that told her was that a child must receive messages, early on, that tell them that they are valued and valuable. This is why you'll see a person, who seems to be wholly-inadequate, achieve unbelievable success; while another with a high IQ, several degrees, and natural creative ability, barely survives. The difference in these two examples is that one has what's called high-emotional intelligence, borne out of a loving upbringing; and the other does not.

A lot was written about Emotional Intelligence back in

the 1980s. It was a new concept to those outside the field of psychology or education. What we learned is that a person's self-view magnifies either a positive, inviting vibration (there's that word again), or a negative one; and thus, this vibration either attracts, or repels. And, we know that no one can make it alone; you need a wide support network of people in the areas that you want to operate, in order to succeed.

The bottom line: realizing decades later you were crippled by child abuse, resulting in low self-awareness, and self-worth, is devastating; because no one can turn back the hands-of-time. However, the "Good News" is as long as you're breathing and have a will to move forward; leaving the past behind, there's the potential that you can live a better tomorrow. Like the line in the hit musical, *Annie*, says: Tomorrow is only a day away! In addition, healing yourself may allow you to become a *beacon* for others who've suffered emotional pain, by example; thus, passing on the joy of forgiveness and reconciliation to others. And, that's the best reward!

My Tea Taste Much Better is designed to help you take that first step *forward*. You're going to feel some strong emotions, but let them come, feel them, get help, and begin anew.

Other Writings by R. Jean Johnson

Epiphanies of the Soul:

52 Life Principles to Live and Love By

Don't Wait, Celebrate Life:

Single Gals Guide to Traveling Solo

These books are available on Amazon.

Website:

Walmart.com/Beaconwear

Email:

beaconwearbooks@gmail.com

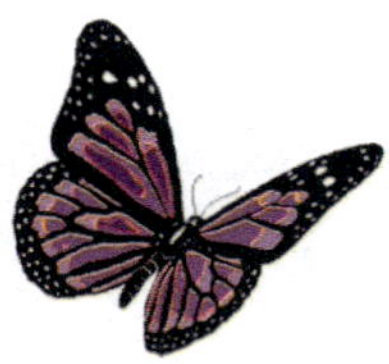

Resources

American Psychological Association (APA)

National Association of Mental Health (NAMI)

988 – National Suicide Hotline

Lifehacks.org – vision board

Pinterest – reconciliation map

Eat these foods to reduce stress and anxiety: Health Essentials, Cleveland Clinic; June 15, 2021

Readers Digest

Daily Beast

Mindfulness Magazine

John Hopkins Hospital – Dr. Swartz

Printed in Great Britain
by Amazon

55691236R00119